The Comprehensive Anti-Inflammatory Diet for Beginners

Reset Inflammation, Heal the Immune System, & Boost Energy by Eating Healthy Food

Linda J. Hebert

1

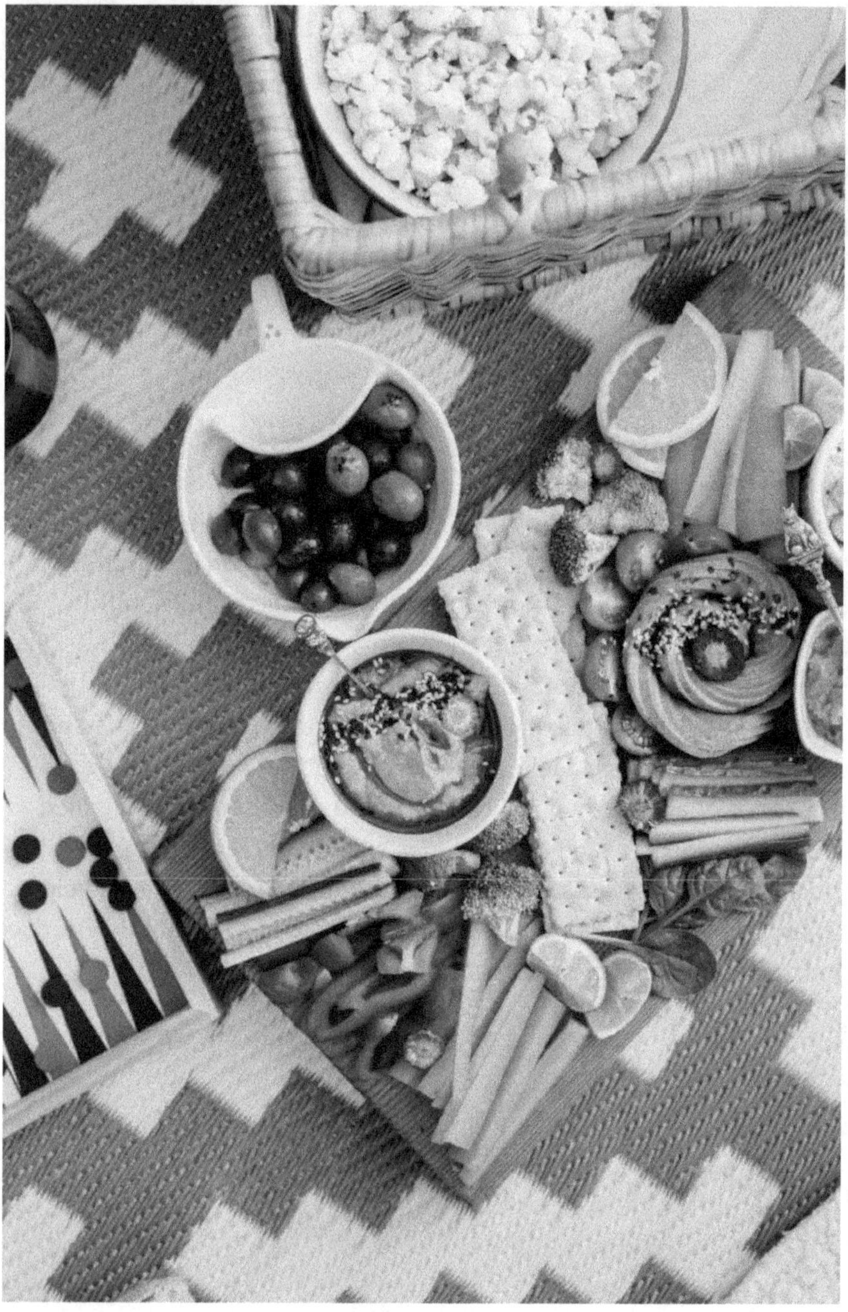

Table of Contents

Introduction

This is the perfect book for reducing inflammation and regulating blood pressure by eating tasty and easy-to-prepare meals!

Start preparing delicious dishes now!

Prawns with Veggies

A wonderful way to organize prawns that each of the family will like

to enjoy. This recipe is perfect for lunch and dinner as

well. Yield: 4 servings

Preparation Time: 15 minutes

Cooking Time: 9 minutes

Ingredients:2 teaspoons coconut

oil 1½ medium onions, sliced

1 tablespoon fresh ginger, grated finely

2 medium green peppers, sliced

3 medium carrots, peeled and sliced

1½ pound pawns, peeled and

deveined 3 garlic cloves, minced

2½ teaspoons curry powder

1½ tablespoons fish sauce

1 cup coconut milk

Water, as required

Salt, to taste

2 tablespoons fresh lime juiceDirections:

1. In a large skillet, melt coconut oil on medium-high heat.

2. Add onion and sauté approximately 1 minute.

3. Add ginger, bell pepper and carrots and stir fry for about 2-3 minutes.

4. Add prawns, garlic, curry powder and fish sauce and stir fry for approximately a few seconds.

5. Add coconut milk plus a little water and stir fry approximately 3-4 minutes.

Nutritional Information per Serving:

Calories: 137, Fat: 4g, Carbohydrates: 19g, Fiber: 6g, Protein: 200g

Pan Fried Squid

A delicious and healthy method to cook the squid for lunchtime.

Ground turmeric gives healthy benefits to squid.

Yield: 2 servings

Preparation Time: 15 minutes Cooking

Time: 13 minutes Ingredients:1 teaspoon

organic olive oil ¼ of yellow onion,

sliced 1-pound squid, cleaned and cut

into rings

¼ teaspoon ground turmeric

Salt, to taste

1 organic egg, beatenDirections:

1. In a skillet, heat oil on medium-high heat.

2. Add onion and sauté for about 4-5 minutes.

3. Add squid rings, turmeric and salt and toss to coat well.

4. Reduce the temperature to medium-low and simmer for

approximately 5 minutes.

5. Add beaten eggs and cook, stirring continuously

approximately 2-3 minutes.

6. Serve hot.

Nutritional Information per Serving:

Calories: 149, Fat: 3g, Carbohydrates: 16g, Fiber: 2g, Protein: 20g

Squid with Veggies

Entertain your household with this particular healthy and satisfying

dish at lunchtime or dinner too. Surely everyone asks to make it again.

Yield: 2 servings

Preparation Time: 20 minutes

Cooking Time: 10 minutes

Ingredients:1 teaspoon extra virgin olive oil

2 carrots, peeled and chopped

2 red bell peppers, seeded and cut into strips

½ of eggplant, chopped

¾ pound squids, cleaned

2 tablespoons fish sauce

1 teaspoon fresh ginger, minced

½ teaspoon paprika

1 cup fresh spinach, chopped

Salt and freshly ground black pepper, to taste

3 small zucchinis, spiralized with Blade CDirections:

1. In a sizable skillet, heat oil on medium heat.

2. Add carrots, bell pepper and eggplant and stir fry

for around 3-4 minutes.

3. Add remaining ingredients except zucchini and cook for

about 1-2 minutes.

4. Stir in spinach and cook for approximately 3-4 minutes.

5. Meanwhile in a very pan of boiling eater, add zucchini

noodles and cook for about 1 minute.

6. Drain well.

7. Transfer the zucchini noodles into two serving bowls.

8. Top with squid mixture and gently stir to blend.

9. Serve immediately.

Nutritional Information per Serving:

Calories: 160, Fat: 4g, Carbohydrates: 21g, Fiber: 7g,
Protein: 23g

Scallops with Veggies

One of a simple and impressive strategy to enjoy scallops and veggies.

This special and simple technique of stir fry gives extra flavor and

texture to this particular dish.

Yield: 1 serving

Preparation Time: 15 minutes

Cooking Time: 9 minutes

Ingredients:½ cup unsalted vegetable broth, divided

1/3 cup carrot, peeled and chopped ¾ cup celery

chopped

1 cup green beans, trimmed and chopped

¾ of green apple, cored and chopped

½ teaspoon fresh ginger herb, grated finely

1 teaspoon ground cardamom

1 teaspoon extra virgin olive oil

4-ouces sea scallops

1 tablespoon walnuts, choppedDirections:

1. In a skillet, heat 3 tablespoons of broth and cook for approximately 4-5 minutes.

2. Stir in green beans, apple, ginger, cardamom and remaining broth and cook approximately 3-4 minutes.

3. Meanwhile in the frying pan, heat oil and cook the scallops for around 2-4 minutes per side.

4. Divide veggie mixture in serving plates.

5. Top with squid and serve.

Nutritional Information per Serving:

Calories: 124, Fat: 5g, Carbohydrates: 16g, Fiber: 8g, Protein: 23g

Scallops with Broccoli

One from the easy meal that's prepared which has a few ingredients.

This delicious meal is often a combo of super healthy ingredients.

Yield: 2 servings

Preparation Time: 15 minutes

Cooking Time: 6 minutes

Ingredients:¼ cup fresh ginger, grated

8 large sea scallops

1 package frozen broccoli, thawed

1 tablespoon coconut oil

Freshly ground black pepper, to tasteDirections:

1. Ina pan of water, add ginger on medium heat.

2. Place scallops in the metal steamer basket and arrange inside the pan of water.

3. Cover and steam for approximately 2-5 minutes.

4. Meanwhile in another pan of boiling water, arrange steamer basket.

5. Add broccoli and boil, covered for approximately 5 minutes.

6. Drain well.

7. In a sizable frying pan, melt coconut oil on medium heat.

8. Add scallops and sear for approximately thirty seconds from each party.

9. Serve the scallops over bed of broccoli.

10. Drizzle having a little ginger water and serve. Nutritional Information per Serving:

Calories: 154, Fat: 4g, Carbohydrates: 13g, Fiber: 9g, Protein: 19g

Spicy Scallops

A wonderfully delicious recipe that will surely impress the scallop

lovers. Combo of spices and veggie paste intensifies the taste of

scallops.

Yield: 3-4 servings

Preparation Time: 15 minutes

Cooking Time: 13 minutes

Ingredients:2 tablespoons coconut milk

½ cup shallot, minced

¼ cup tomato paste

2 teaspoons fresh ginger paste

2 teaspoons garlic paste

½ teaspoon garam masala

¼ teaspoon ground cinnamon

¼ teaspoon ground cumin

Pinch of red pepper cayenne

Salt, to taste

1-pound sea scallops

8-ounce plain Greek yogurt, whipped

Chopped fresh cilantro, for garnishingDirections:

1. In a large skillet, melt coconut oil on medium-high heat

2. Add shallots and sauté approximately 2-3 minutes.

3. Add remaining ingredients except scallops, yogurt

and cilantro and cook for about 3-5 minutes.

4. Stir in scallops and yogurt and cook approximately

5 minutes.

5. Serve hot using the garnishing of cilantro.

Nutritional Information per Serving:

Calories: 217, Fat: 2g, Carbohydrates: 11g, Fiber: 5g,
Protein: 10g

Deep Fried Kingfish

A simple deep-fried fish recipe with all the abundance delicious

flavors. This recipe prepares fish with crispiness about the outside and

soft inside

Yield: 4 servings

Preparation Time: 15 minutes

Cooking Time: 8 minutes

Ingredients:½ teaspoon ginger paste

½ teaspoon garlic paste

2 tablespoons chickpea flour

2 teaspoons turmeric powder

1 teaspoon ground coriander

1 teaspoon red chili powder

½ teaspoon garam

masala Salt, to taste

Water, as required

1-pound kingfisher fillets

Olive oil, as necessary for deep fryingDirections:

1. In a large bowl, add all of the ingredients except the fish and oil and mix till a paste form.

2. Add the fish fillets and coat using the paste generously.

3. Refrigerate to marinate for approximately 1 hour.

4. In a substantial deep skillet, heat oil on medium-high heat.

5. Add fish fillets and fry for about 3-4 minutes per side or till desired doneness.

6. Transfer onto a paper towel lined plate to drain. Nutritional Information per Serving:

Calories: 160, Fat: 4g, Carbohydrates: 17g, Fiber: 5g, Protein: 24g

Spicy Kingfish

Enjoy an exclusive recipe of fried fish that's constructed with simple

spice combo. Combo of spices makes this fried fish very tasty.

Yield: 2 servings

Preparation Time: 15 minutes

Cooking Time: 10 minutes

Ingredients:1 teaspoon dried unsweetened coconut

1 teaspoon cumin seeds

1 teaspoon fennel seeds

1 teaspoon peppercorns

10 curry leaves

½ teaspoon ground turmeric

1½ teaspoons fresh ginger, grated finely

1 garlic herb, minced Salt, to taste

1 tablespoon fresh lime juice

4 (4-ounce) kingfish steaks

1 tbsp. olive oil

1 lime wedgeDirections:

1. Heat a surefire skillet on low heat.

2. Add coconut, cumin seeds, fennel seeds, peppercorns and

curry leaves and cook, stirring continuously for about

1 minute.

3. Remove in the heat and let it cool completely.

4. In a spice grinder, add the spice mixture and turmeric

and grind rill powdered finely.

5. Transfer the mixture in to a large bowl with

ginger, garlic, salt and lime juice and mix well.

6. Add fish fillets and cat while using mixture evenly.

7. Refrigerate to marinate approximately 3 hours.

8. In a big nonstick skillet, heat oil on medium heat.

9. Add the fish fillets and cook for approximately 3-

5 minutes per side or till desired doneness.

10. Transfer onto a paper towel lined plate to drain.

11. Serve with lime wedges.

Nutritional Information per Serving:

Calories: 149, Fat: 6g, Carbohydrates: 20g, Fiber: 2g, Protein: 21g

Gingered Tilapia

One with the super-fast and straightforward recipe of the healthy fish.

This tilapia is seasoned deliciously having a few ingredients.

Yield: 5 servings

Preparation Time: 15 minutes

Cooking Time: 6 minutes

Ingredients:2 tablespoons coconut oil

5 tilapia fillets

3 garlic cloves, minced

2 tablespoons unsweetened coconut, shredded

4-ounce freshly ground ginger

2 tablespoons coconut aminos

8 scallions, choppedDirections:

1. In a large skillet, melt coconut oil on medium heat.

2. Add tilapia fillets and cook for around 2 minutes.

3. Flip the inside and add garlic, coconut and ginger and cook for about 1 minute.

4. Add coconut aminos and cook for around 1 minute.

5. Add scallion and cook for approximately 1-2 minute more.

6. Serve immediately.

Nutritional Information per Serving:

Calories: 135, Fat: 3g, Carbohydrates: 2g, Fiber 5g, Protein: 26g

Spicy Salmon

A lip-smacking recipe of healthiest salmon. This aromatic and spicy

marinade creates a rich and deep flavor inside

salmon. Yield: 4 servings

Preparation Time: 15 minutes

Cooking Time: 7 minutes

Ingredients:Salt, to taste

2 small onions, chopped

2 large garlic cloves, chopped

1 (1-inch) piece fresh ginger, chopped

1 teaspoon ground turmeric

2 teaspoons red chili powder

Salt and freshly ground black pepper, to

taste 2 tablespoons fresh lemon juice 4

salmon steaks

Coconut oil, as required for shallow fryingDirections:

1. In a food processor, add all ingredients except salmon and oil and pulse till smooth.

2. Transfer the mix right into a bowl.

3. Add steaks and coat with marinade generously.

4. Refrigerate to marinate for overnight.

5. In a large skillet, melt coconut oil on medium-high heat.

6. Add salmon fillet, skin-side up and cook for approximately 4 minutes.

7. Flip the medial side and cook for approximately 3 minutes.

8. Transfer onto a paper towel lined plate to drain.

9. Serve with lemon wedges.

Nutritional Information per Serving:

Calories: 177, Fat: 3g, Carbohydrates: 17g, Fiber: 6g, Protein: 19g

Crispy Salmon

An amazing recipe of crispy salmon. This fried crispy salmon fish will

likely be an excellent choice for any pot-luck party or meet up.

Yield: 4 servings

Preparation Time: 15 minutes

Cooking Time: 12 minutes

Ingredients:1 teaspoon garlic powder

1 teaspoon ground coriander

2 teaspoons red pepper flakes, crushed

1 teaspoon red chili powder

Salt and freshly ground black pepper, to taste

2 tablespoons fresh lemon juice 4 salmon

steaks

1 cup chickpea flour

Olive oil, as essential for deep fryingDirections:

1. In a sizable bowl, mix together all ingredients

except salmon, chickpea flour and oil.

2. Add salmon steaks and coat with mixture evenly.

3. Refrigerate to marinate for around 3-4 hours.

4. In a shallow dish, place chickpea flour.

5. In a skillet, heat oil on medium-high heat.

6. Coat the salmon steaks with flour evenly.

7. Fry the salmon fillets approximately 5-6 minutes per side.

8. Transfer onto a paper towel lined plate to

drain. Nutritional Information per Serving:

Calories: 168, Fat: 5g, Carbohydrates: 19g, Fiber: 2g, Protein: 24g

Salmon with Cabbage

A special recipe of healthy salmon with crunchy cabbage. Salmon and

cabbage produce a really delicious combo for

supper. Yield: 4 servings

Preparation Time: 15 minutes

Cooking Time: 10 minutes

Ingredients:1 (1-inch) piece fresh ginger, grated

finely 2 tablespoons taw honey

1 tablespoon freshly squeezed lemon juice

1 tablespoon Dijon mustard

4 tablespoons organic olive oil, divided

4 (8-ounce) salmon fillets

1 small head cabbage, sliced thinly

1 garlic clove, minced

1 tablespoon sesame seeds

Freshly ground black pepper, to taste

4 scallions, choppedDirections:

1. In a bowl, mix together ginger, honey, fresh lemon juice

and Dijon mustard. Keep aside.

2. In a sizable nonstick skillet, heat 1 tablespoon of oil on medium-high heat.

3. Add salmon and cook for around 3-4 minutes per side.

4. Place the honey mixture over salmon fillets evenly and immediately remove from heat.

5. Cover and make aside till serving.

6. Meanwhile in another skillet, heat 2 tablespoons of oil on medium heat.

7. Add cabbage and stir fry for approximately 3-4 minutes.

8. Add remaining oil and stir fry for around 5 minutes.

9. Add garlic, sesame seeds and black pepper and cook for about 1 minute.

10. Place salmon over cabbage and serve with garnishing of scallion.

Nutritional Information per Serving:

Calories: 150, Fat: 6g, Carbohydrates: 22g, Fiber: 8g, Protein: 21g

Salmon with Vegetables

One from the delicious and wonderful plate to your family. This plate

is often a great mixture of nutritious and colorful ingredients.

Yield: 1 serving

Preparation Time: 20 minutes

Cooking Time: 19 minutes

Ingredients:5 teaspoons extra virgin olive oil, divided

1 teaspoon ground turmeric 1 teaspoon paprika

Salt and freshly ground black pepper, to taste

1 (4-ounce) salmon fillet

1 purple baby carrot, cut lengthwise

1 yellow carrot, cut lengthwise

1 orange carrot, cut lengthwise

3 French beans, chopped

3 button mushrooms, slicedDirections:

1. In a bowl, mix together 2 teaspoons of oil, turmeric,

paprika, salt and black pepper.

2. Add salmon and coat using the oil mixture evenly. Keep aside.

3. In a pan of boiling water, add French beans and carrots and cook for about 3 minutes.

4. Drain well.

5. In a nonstick skillet, heat 2 teaspoons of oil on medium heat.

6. Add mushroom and a pinch of salt and black pepper and stir fry for or about 5-6 minutes.

7. Add the drained vegetables and stir fry approximately 2 minutes.

8. Transfer the vegetables onto a plate and loosely, cover having a foil paper to hold warm.

9. In a similar skillet, heat remaining oil on medium heat.

10. Add salmon filler, skin-side down and cook for approximately 3-5 minutes.

11. Change the inside and cook for approximately 2-3 minutes.

12. Place salmon over vegetables and

serve. Nutritional Information per Serving:

Calories: 162, Fat: 5g, Carbohydrates: 15g, Fiber: 10g, Protein: 20g

Basa with Mushroom & Bell Pepper

One from the great recipes on your dining room table. Simple

seasoning with fish sauce and coconut aminos adds an excellent flavor

in this meal.

Yield: 2 servings

Preparation Time: 15 minutes

Cooking Time: 18 minutes

Ingredients:1 (8-ounce) basa fish fillet, cubed

¼ teaspoon ginger paste

¼ teaspoon garlic paste

1 teaspoon red chili powder

Salt, to taste

1 tablespoon coconut vinegar

1 tablespoon extra-virgin organic olive oil, divided

½ cup fresh mushrooms, sliced

1 small onion, quartered

¼ cup red bell pepper, seeded and cubed

¼ cup yellow bell pepper, seeded and

cubed 2-3 scallions, chopped

1 teaspoon fish sauceDirections:

1. In a bowl, mix together fish, ginger, garlic, chili powder

and salt whilst aside for around twenty minutes.

2. In a nonstick skillet, heat 1 teaspoon of oil
on medium high heat.

3. Sear the fish for about 5-6 minutes or till golden

coming from all sides.

4. In another skillet, heat remaining oil on medium heat.

5. Add mushrooms and onion and stir fry for about 5-

7 minutes.

6. Add bell pepper and fish and stir fry for about 2 minutes.

7. Add scallion and fish sauce and stir fry for bout 1-

2 minutes.

8. Serve hot.

Nutritional Information per Serving:

Calories: 170, Fat: 5g, Carbohydrates: 19g, Fiber: 11g,
Protein: 25g

Haddock with Swiss Chard

A light but healthy meal for warm summer days. This meal is

prepared with ingredients which can be easily available in your

pantry.

Yield: 1 serving

Preparation Time: 15 minutes

Cooking Time: 10 minutes

Ingredients:2 tablespoons coconut oil,

divided 2 minced garlic cloves

2 teaspoons fresh ginger, grated finely

1 haddock fillet

Salt and freshly ground black pepper, to taste

2 cups Swiss chard, chopped roughly 1

teaspoon coconut aminosDirections:

1. In a skillet, melt 1 tablespoon of coconut oil on

medium heat.

2. Add garlic and ginger and sauté approximately 1 minute.

3. Add haddock fillet and sprinkle with salt and black pepper.

4. Cook approximately 3-5 minutes per side or till desired doneness.

5. Meanwhile in another skillet, melt remaining coconut oil on medium heat.

6. Add Swiss chard and coconut aminos and cook for around 5-10 minutes.

7. Serve the salmon fillet over Swiss chard.

Nutritional Information per Serving:

Calories: 176, Fat: 4g, Carbohydrates: 17g, Fiber: 4g, Protein: 21g

Snapper with Carrot & Broccoli

A great dish of fish and veggies with sweet and sour flavors. Snapper

fillets come up with a delicious accompaniment to healthy veggies.

Yield: 2 servings

Preparation Time: 15 minutes

Cooking Time: 6 minutes

Ingredients:2½ tbsps. essential olive oil, divided

1 teaspoon red curry paste Salt, to taste

2 skinless snapper fillets

2 teaspoons coconut oil, divided

½ tablespoon fresh ginger, sliced thinly

10 baby carrots, peeled and halved

1 tablespoon fish sauce

1½ tablespoons freshly squeezed lemon juice,

divided 1 teaspoon organic honey

2 cups broccoli florets

Freshly ground black pepper, to taste

1 garlic clove, mincedDirections:

1. In a bowl, mix together 2 tablespoons of essential olive oil, curry paste and salt.

2. Add snapper fillets and rub with oil mixture evenly. Keep aside for about 5-10 min.

3. In a small skillet, melt 1 teaspoon of coconut oil on medium heat.

4. Add ginger and carrots and stir fry for around 2 minutes.

5. Add fish sauce, 1 tablespoon of fresh lemon juice, honey and black pepper and stir fry approximately 2-3 minutes.

6. Meanwhile in another skillet, heat remaining olive oil on medium heat.

7. Add snapper fillets and cook for about 3 minutes from both sides.

8. Drizzle with remaining lemon juice.

9. Meanwhile in a pan of boiling water add broccoli and cook for around 2 minutes.

10. Drain well.

11. In a similar pan, melt remaining coconut oil on medium heat.

12. Add garlic and sauté for around 1 minute.

13. Add broccoli and toss to coat well.

14. Serve snapper fillets with carrots and broccoli. Nutritional Information per Serving:

Calories: 169, Fat: 5g, Carbohydrates: 17g, Fiber: 5g, Protein: 26g

Citrus Poached Salmon

An absolutely great way to prepare salmon fish.
Fresh orange juice

adds a delish citrus touch in salmon.

Yield: 3 servings

Preparation Time: 15 minutes

Cooking Time: 12 minutes

Ingredients:3 garlic cloves, crushed

1½ teaspoons fresh ginger, grated finely

1/3 cup fresh orange juice

3 tablespoons coconut aminos

3 (6-ounce) salmon filletsDirections:

1. Ina bowl, mix together all ingredients except salmon.

2. In the bottom of your large pan, squeeze salmon fillet.

3. Place the ginger mixture in the salmon and aside for

about 15 minutes.

4. Place the pan on high heat and convey to your boil.

5. Reduce the heat to low and simmer, covered for about
10-

12 minutes or till desired doneness.

Nutritional Information per Serving:

Calories: 179, Fat: 5.2g, Carbohydrates: 17.2g, Fiber: 4g, Protein: 27g

Steamed Snapper Parcel

A delicious snapper recipe with extraordinary flavors. This steamed

fish is delicious and so healthful at the same

time. Yield: 2 servings

Preparation Time: 15 minutes Cooking

Time: 10 minutes Ingredients:2

tablespoons garlic, minced 1 tablespoon

fresh turmeric, grated finely 1

tablespoon fresh ginger, grated finely 2

tablespoons fresh lime juice 2

tablespoons coconut aminos

2 tablespoons essential olive oil

1 bunch fresh cilantro, chopped

2 (6-ounce) snapper filletsDirections:

1. In a food processor, add garlic, turmeric, ginger, lime

juice, coconut aminos and extra virgin olive oil and

pulse till smooth.

2. Transfer a combination in the bowl with cilantro and

mix well.

3. Add snapper fillets and coat using the

mixture generously.

4. Place each fish fillet in the foil paper and wrap the paper

to create a parcel.

5. Arrange a steamer basket inside a pan of boiling water.

6. Place the parcels in steamer basket.

7. Cover and steam for about 10 min.

Nutritional Information per Serving:

Calories: 155, Fat: 4g, Carbohydrates: 20g, Fiber: 2g,
Protein: 26g

Broiled Spicy Salmon

A fantastic dinner that is prepared within 20 minutes. The blending of

yogurt and spices makes the salmon flavorful and moist.

Yield: 4 servings

Preparation Time: 15 minutes

Cooking Time: 14 minutes

Ingredients:¼ cup low- Fat plain Greek yogurt

½ teaspoon ground coriander

½ teaspoon ground turmeric

½ teaspoon ground ginger

¼ tsp cayenne pepper

Salt and freshly ground black pepper, to taste

4 (6-ounce) skinless salmon filletsDirections:

1. Heat the broiler of the oven. Grease a broiler pan.

2. In a bowl, mix together all ingredients except the salmon.

3. Arrange salmon fillets onto prepared broiler pan inside a

single layer.

4. Place the yogurt mixture over each fillet evenly.

5. Broil approximately 12-14 minutes.

6. Serve immediately.

Nutritional Information per Serving:

Calories: 163, Fat: 3g, Carbohydrates: 15g, Fiber: 6g, Protein: 20g

Broiled Sweet & Tangy Salmon

One from the most enjoyable dish of salmon. This marinade enhances

the flavor of nutritious salmon greatly.

Yield: 3 servings

Preparation Time: 15 minutes

Cooking Time: 12 minutes

Ingredients:2 garlic cloves, crushed

2 tablespoons fresh ginger grated finely

2 tablespoons organic honey

2 tablespoons coconut aminos

2 tablespoons fresh lime juice

3 tablespoons olive oil

3 tablespoons sesame oil

2 tablespoons black sesame seeds

1 tablespoon white sesame seeds

1-pound boneless salmon fillets

1/3 cup scallion, choppedDirections:

1. In a baking dish, mix together all ingredients except the

salmon. And scallion.

2. Add salmon and coat with mixture generously.

3. Refrigerate to marinate for about 40-45 minutes.

4. Preheat the broiler of oven and arrange the rack inside top in the oven.

5. Place the baking dish inside the oven and broil for approximately 10-12 minutes.

6. In serving platter, put the salmon and top with all the pan sauce.

7. Serve while using garnishing of scallion.

Nutritional Information per Serving:

Calories: 155, Fat: 5g, Carbohydrates: 22g, Fiber: 5g, Protein: 22g

Baked Sweet Lemony Salmon

A simple recipe that makes salmon really delicious and filling. Surely

this salmon recipe can be family favorite.

Yield: 2 servings

Preparation Time: 15 minutes

Cooking Time: 12 minutes

Ingredients:2 (8-ounce) salmon fillets

½ teaspoon organic honey and even more for

drizzling 1/3 teaspoon ground turmeric, divided

Freshly ground black pepper, to taste

2 large lemon slicesDirections:

1. In a zip lock bag, add salmon, ½ teaspoon of honey, ¼

teaspoon of turmeric and black pepper.

2. Seal the bag and shake to coat well.

3. Refrigerate to marinate for around 1 hour.

4. Preheat the oven to 40 degrees F.

5. Transfer the salmon fillets onto a cookie sheet in the

single layer.

6. Cover the fillets with marinade.

7. Place the salmon fillets, skin-side up and bake for around 6 minutes.

8. Carefully, customize the side of fillets.

9. Sprinkle with remaining turmeric and black pepper evenly.

10. Place 1 lemon slice over each fillet and drizzle with honey.

11. Bake for approximately 6 minutes.

Nutritional Information per Serving:

Calories: 171, Fat: 3g, Carbohydrates: 15g, Fiber: 2g, Protein: 21g

Baked parsley Salmon

A recipe of tasty salmon that requires no fuss for preparation. This

meal is prepared with only 5 ingredients.

Yield: 3-4 servings

Preparation Time: 15 minutes Cooking

Time: 20 or so minutes Ingredients:16-

24-ounce salmon fillets 2 tablespoons

coconut oil, melted 3 tablespoons fresh

parsley, minced

¼ teaspoon ginger powder

Salt, to tasteDirections:

1. Preheat the oven to 400 degrees F. Grease a substantial

baking dish.

2. Arrange the salmon fillets into prepared baking dish in

a single layer.

3. Drizzle with coconut oil and sprinkle with parsley,

ginger powder and salt.

4. Bake for about 15-twenty or so minutes.

Nutritional Information per Serving:

Calories: 168, Fat: 5g, Carbohydrates: 14g, Fiber: 7g, Protein: 20g

Baked Walnut & Lemon Crusted Salmon

A restaurant quality recipe that you can prepare at home easily.

Walnut gives a really nice crunchy crust for the salmon.

Yield: 4 servings

Preparation Time: 15 minutes

Cooking Time: 20 minutes

Ingredients:1 cup walnuts

1 tablespoon fresh dill, chopped

2 tablespoons fresh lemon rind, grated

½ teaspoon garlic salt

Freshly ground black pepper, to taste

1 tbsp. olive oil

3-4 tablespoons Dijon mustard

4 (3-ounce) salmon fillets

4 teaspoons fresh lemon juiceDirections:

1. Preheat the oven to 350 degrees F. Line a

substantial baking sheet with parchment paper.

2. In a mixer, add walnuts and pulse till hoped roughly.

3. Add dill, lemon rind, garlic salt, black pepper and oil and pulse till a crumbly mixture form.

4. Place the salmon fillets, skin-side on to prepared baking sheet in a very single layer.

5. Coat the surface of each salmon fillet with Dijon mustard

evenly.

6. Place the walnut mixture over each fillet evenly and gently, press into the surface of salmon.

7. Bake for about 15-20 min.

8. Serve with the drizzling of fresh lemon juice.

Nutritional Information per Serving:

Calories: 173, Fat: 8g, Carbohydrates: 2g, Fiber: 2g, Protein: 22g

Baked Crispy Cod

One with the fantastic way to arrange cod for dinner within 20

minutes. This recipe adds a bright yellow color to delicious cod.

Yield: 2-4 servings

Preparation Time: 15 minutes

Cooking Time: 15 minutes

Ingredients:1 green bell pepper, seeded and

sliced 2 large eggs

1/3 cup blanched almond flour

¼ teaspoon dried dill weed, crushed

½ teaspoon garlic powder

1/8 teaspoon ground turmeric

Freshly ground black pepper, to

taste 1½ pound cod fillets

Chopped fresh chives, for garnishingDirections:

1. Preheat the oven to 350 degrees F. Line a large

rimmed baking dish with parchment paper.

2. Arrange the bell pepper slices into prepared baking dish.

3. In a shallow dish, crack the eggs and brat well.

4. In another shallow dish, mix together almond flour, dill weed, garlic powder, turmeric and black pepper.

5. Coat the cod fillets in egg and then roll into flour mixture

evenly.

6. Place the cod fillets over bell pepper slices.

7. Bake for approximately fifteen minutes.

8. Serve with all the garnishing of chives.

Nutritional Information per Serving:

Calories: 170, Fat: 5g, Carbohydrates: 17g, Fiber: 6g, Protein: 26g

Baked Cheesy Salmon

A great addition inside your seafood menu list. Topping of cheddar

cheese brings a delish twist in baked salmon recipes.

Yield: 4 servings

Preparation Time: 15 minutes

Cooking Time: 25 minutes

Ingredients:2 garlic cloves, crushed

1 teaspoon dried dill weed, crushed

Salt and freshly ground black pepper, to taste

2-pounds salmon fillets

1 cup cheddar cheese, shredded

6 scallions, choppedDirections:

1. Preheat the oven to 450 degrees F.

2. In a bowl, mix together garlic, dill weed, salt and

black pepper.

3. Sprinkle the salmon fillets with garlic mixture evenly.

4. Arrange the salmon fillets over a big foil paper and

fold to seal.

5. Place the salmon parcel in a very baking sheet and bake approximately twenty minutes.

6. Now, unfold the parcel and top the salmon fillets with cheese and scallions.

7. Bake for about 5 minutes.

Nutritional Information per Serving:

Calories: 115, Fat: 3.4g, Carbohydrates: 2.9g, Fiber: 0.7g, Protein: 28.3g

Grilled Sweet & Tangy Salmon

A super-fast and simple meal for busy weekends. Definitely whole

family will like to enjoy this sweet and tangy

salmon. Yield: 4 servings

Preparation Time: 15 minutes

Cooking Time: 15 minutes

Ingredients:1 scallion, chopped

1 teaspoon garlic powder 1

teaspoon ground ginger

¼ cup organic honey

1/3 cup fresh orange juice

1/3 cup coconut aminos

1½ pound salmon filletsDirections:

1. In a zip lock bag, add all ingredients and seal the bag.

2. Shake the bag to coat the mix with salmon.

3. Refrigerate for around thirty minutes, flipping occasionally.

4. Preheat the grill to medium heat. Grease the grill grate.

5. Remove the salmon from your bag, reserving the marinade.

6. Grill for around 10 minutes.

7. Coat the fillets with reserved marinade and grill for 5 minutes more.

Nutritional Information per Serving:

Calories: 206.8, Fat: 7.6g, Carbohydrates: 20.6g, Fiber: 0.5g, Protein:

26.5g

Grilled Salmon with Peach & Onion

One with the best recipe for barbecue parties. This healthy dinner

plate is packed using the flavors of healthy salmon and sweet peach.

Yield: 4 servings

Preparation Time: 15 minutes

Cooking Time: 12 minutes

Ingredients:4 salmon steaks

Salt and freshly ground black pepper, to taste

3 peaches, pitted and cut into wedges 2

medium red onions, cut into wedges

1 tablespoon fresh ginger, minced

1 teaspoon fresh thyme leaves, minced

3 tablespoons essential olive oil

1 tablespoon balsamic vinegarDirections:

1. Preheat the grill to medium heat. Grease the grill grate.

2. Sprinkle the salmon with salt and black pepper evenly.

3. In a bowl, add peach, onion, salt and black pepper and

toss to coat well.

4. Grill the salmon steaks for approximately 5-6 minutes.

5. Now, place peaches and onions on grill with salmon steaks.

6. Grill the salmon for about 5-6 minutes per side.

7. Grill the peaches and onion for around 3-4 minutes per side.

8. Meanwhile in a bowl, add remaining ingredients and mix till a smooth paste form.

9. Place ginger mixture over salmon filets evenly and serve with peaches and onions.

Nutritional Information per Serving:

Calories: 185, Fat: 4g, Carbohydrates: 24g, Fiber: 4g, Protein: 30.3g

Grilled Spicy Salmon

A family friendly fish recipe for weekends. Combo of orange juice and

spices adds a delicious richness in salmon.

Yield: 6-8 servings

Preparation Time: 15 minutes

Cooking Time: 6-10 minutes

Ingredients:½ tablespoon ground ginger

½ tablespoon ground coriander

½ tablespoon ground cumin

½ teaspoon paprika

¼ tsp red pepper

cayenne Salt, to taste

1 tablespoon fresh orange juice

1 tablespoon coconut oil, melted 1½-

2-pound salmon filletsDirections:

1. In a big bowl, add all ingredients except salmon and mix till a paste form.

2. Add salmon and coat with mixture generously.

3. Refrigerate to marinate for approximately thirty minutes.

4. Preheat the propane gas grill to high heat using the lid closed not less than 10 minutes.

5. Grease the grill and place the salmon fillets, skin-side down.

6. Cover with all the lid and grill approximately 3 minutes.

7. Flip the medial side and cover while using lid and grill for around 3 minutes more.

Nutritional Information per Serving:

Calories: 193, Fat: 6g, Carbohydrates: 17g, Fiber: 6g, Protein: 32g

Shrimp Curry

Delicious anti-inflammatory shrimp curry

recipes. Yield: 4 servings

Preparation Time: 15 minutes

Cooking Time: 18 minutes

Ingredients:2 tablespoons peanut oil

½ sweet onion, minced

2 minced garlic cloves

1½ teaspoons ground turmeric

1 teaspoon ground cumin

1 teaspoon ground ginger

1 teaspoon paprika

½ teaspoon red chili powder 1

(14-ounce) can coconut milk

1 (14 ½-ounce) can chopped tomatoes

Salt, to taste

1-pound cooked shrimp, peeled and deveined

2 tablespoons fresh cilantro, choppedDirections:

1. In a big skillet, heat oil on medium heat.

2. Add onion and sauté approximately 5 minutes.

3. Reduce the temperature to low.

4. Add garlic and spices and sauté for around 1 minute.

5. Add coconut milk, tomatoes and salt and simmer

for about 10 min, stirring occasionally.

6. Stir in the shrimp and cilantro and simmer

approximately 1-2 minutes.

Nutritional Information per Serving:

Calories: 216, Fat: 12.1g, Carbohydrates: 10. g, Fiber: 3g,
Protein: 23g

Rockfish Curry

A fish curry with mild spicy touch. This wonderfully delicious meal is

actually enjoyable for dinner parties too.

Yield: 8 servings

Preparation Time: 15 minutes

Cooking Time: 30 minutes

Ingredients:2-pound rockfish

¾ teaspoon ground turmeric, divided

Salt, to taste

2 tablespoons coconut oil

12 pearl onions, halved

2 medium red onions, sliced thinly

2 Serrano peppers, halved

40 small leaves, divided

1 (½-inch) piece fresh ginger,

minced Freshly ground black pepper,

to taste ¼ cup water

1½ (14-ounce) cans coconut milk, divided

1 teaspoon using apple cider vinegarDirections:

1. In a bowl, season the fish with ¼ teaspoon with the turmeric and salt whilst aside.

2. In a sizable skillet, melt coconut oil on medium heat.

3. Add pearl onions, red onions, ginger, Serrano peppers and 20 curry leaves and sauté approximately 15 minutes.

4. Add ginger, remaining turmeric, salt and black pepper and sauté for approximately 2 minutes.

5. Transfer half of the mixture in to a bowl whilst aside.

6. Add remaining curry leaves, fish fillets, water and 1 can of coconut milk and cook for approximately 2 minutes.

7. Now cook, covered approximately 5 minutes.

8. Add apple cider vinegar and remaining half can of coconut milk and cook for around 3-5 minutes or till done completely.

9. Serve hot using the topping of reserved onion mixture.

Nutritional Information per Serving:

Calories: 179, Fat: 12g, Carbohydrates: 16g, Fiber: 8g, Protein: 27g

CPSIA information can be obtained
at www.ICGtesting.com
Printed in the USA
BVHW090630270421
605864BV00004B/789